CIALIS

Basic Guide On How To Boost Libido, Get Hard ,Stay Healthy , Stay Active Using Cialis.

Peter Park

Table of Contents

Chapter1 3

    Introduction to cialis 3

Chapter2 16

    Dosage of cialis 16

Chapter3 25

    How does cialis works 25

    The end 30

Chapter 1

Introduction to cialis

Cialis is a medication primarily used to treat erectile dysfunction (ED) and symptoms of benign prostatic hyperplasia (BPH), which is an enlarged prostate. Its active ingredient is tadalafil, which belongs to a class of drugs called phosphodiesterase type 5 (PDE5) inhibitors.

Cialis works by relaxing the smooth muscles in the blood vessels, allowing for increased blood flow to certain areas of the body, particularly the penis, which helps to achieve and maintain an erection during sexual stimulation. It does not lead to spontaneous erections and requires sexual arousal to be effective.

In addition to treating ED, Cialis is also prescribed in a lower dose as a daily treatment for BPH and ED/BPH when these conditions occur together. It's important to note that Cialis should only be used under the supervision of a healthcare provider, as it may interact with other medications and could have side effects.

effects.

Uses of cialis

Cialis, or its generic counterpart tadalafil, has several uses:

Treatment of Erectile Dysfunction (ED): Cialis is primarily prescribed to treat erectile dysfunction, a condition characterized by the inability to achieve or maintain an erection sufficient for sexual intercourse. It helps increase blood flow to the penis, facilitating erections when a man is sexually stimulated.

Treatment of Benign Prostatic Hyperplasia (BPH): Cialis is also approved for the treatment of benign prostatic hyperplasia, a condition in which the prostate gland becomes enlarged, leading to urinary symptoms such as frequent urination, difficulty starting or maintaining urination, weak urine stream, or the feeling of incomplete bladder emptying. Cialis helps relax the smooth muscles in the prostate and bladder, improving urinary symptoms.

Treatment of Both Erectile Dysfunction and BPH: In some cases, Cialis may be prescribed for both erectile dysfunction and benign prostatic hyperplasia simultaneously, as it addresses both conditions.

Treatment of Pulmonary Arterial Hypertension (PAH): In some countries, Cialis is approved for the treatment of pulmonary arterial hypertension, a type of high blood pressure that affects the arteries in the lungs and the right side of the heart. Cialis helps relax the blood vessels in the lungs, reducing the workload on the heart and improving exercise capacity.

Off-Label Uses: Cialis may sometimes be prescribed off-label for other conditions, such as Raynaud's phenomenon (a condition characterized by reduced blood flow to the fingers and toes), high-altitude pulmonary edema (fluid accumulation in the lungs at high altitudes), or for enhancing exercise performance in athletes. However, the effectiveness and safety of Cialis for these uses may vary, and it's essential to consult with a healthcare provider before using it off-label.

Chapter 2

Dosage of cialis

The dosage of Cialis (tadalafil) can vary depending on the individual's needs, medical condition, and response to treatment. It's essential to follow your healthcare provider's instructions regarding dosage. Here are the typical dosage options for Cialis:

As Needed Dosing for Erectile Dysfunction (ED):

The usual starting dose is 10 mg taken prior to anticipated sexual activity.

Depending on how well the medication works

and how well it is tolerated, the dose may be increased to 20 mg or decreased to 5 mg. Your healthcare provider will determine the appropriate dose for you.

Cialis is typically taken as needed, with a maximum frequency of once per day.

Daily Dosing for Erectile Dysfunction (ED):

For some individuals, especially those who anticipate frequent sexual activity (more than twice per week), a lower daily dose of Cialis may be prescribed.

The recommended dose for daily use is 2.5 mg to 5 mg taken once daily at approximately the same time each day.

This dosing regimen allows for more spontaneous sexual activity without the need to plan for medication timing.

Treatment of Benign Prostatic Hyperplasia (BPH):

The usual dose for the treatment of benign prostatic hyperplasia is 5 mg once daily, regardless of sexual activity.

Cialis for BPH can be taken with or without food.

Combined Treatment for Erectile Dysfunction and BPH:

In cases where a patient has both erectile dysfunction and benign prostatic hyperplasia, Cialis may be prescribed at a dose of 5 mg once daily.

Treatment of Pulmonary Arterial Hypertension (PAH):

The dosage for the treatment of pulmonary arterial hypertension is typically higher and varies depending on the severity of the condition and individual response. This is usually determined by a healthcare provider experienced in managing PAH.

Chapter 3

How does cialis works

When a man is sexually stimulated, nitric oxide is released into the penis. Nitric oxide stimulates an enzyme called guanylate cyclase, which increases levels of cyclic guanosine monophosphate (cGMP). This results in the relaxation of smooth muscles in the penis, allowing for increased blood flow.

Increased Blood Flow: The relaxation of smooth muscles and increased levels of cGMP lead to dilation of blood vessels in the penis. This dilation allows more blood to flow into the penis, causing it to become erect.

PDE5 Inhibition: Cialis works by inhibiting the enzyme PDE5. PDE5 is responsible for breaking down cGMP, so by inhibiting PDE5, Cialis helps to maintain higher levels of cGMP in the penis. This prolongs the effects of nitric oxide, leading to prolonged relaxation of smooth muscles and increased blood flow, which in turn helps to sustain an erection.

Duration of Action: One of the key advantages of Cialis compared to other ED medications like Viagra is its longer duration of action. While Viagra typically lasts for about 4-6 hours, Cialis can remain effective for up to 36 hours. This longer duration of action has earned Cialis the nickname "the weekend pill."

The end

Made in the USA
Columbia, SC
08 August 2024